Arthritis Diet:

Anti-inflammatory Diet for Arthritis Pain Relief

Table of Contents

Additionally, the information in the following pages is intended only for informational purposes and should thus be thought of as universal. As befitting its nature, it is presented without assurance regarding its prolonged validity or interim quality. Trademarks that are mentioned are done without written consent and can in no way be considered an endorsement from the trademark holder.

Chapter 1: Introduction

Congratulations on purchasing the *Arthritis Diet* and thank you for doing so.

If you have purchased this book, it's possible you or a loved one have symptoms of arthritis and joint pain. Maybe you even have inflammation and been diagnosed with an inflammatory disease. If that's the case, we can understand how hard that is for you, and we sympathize with you. This book is a great introductory read to learn about the symptoms of joint pain and arthritis, as well as how inflammation affects the body. It explains these conditions so you can become familiar with them and can easily recognize symptoms that might be plaguing you. Whether you are experiencing pain, stiffness of the joints, or having limited motor function, arthritis can affect every individual differently. It can be a struggle trying to figure out how to work around the pain as your normal daily routine is interrupted. Whether you are elderly or not, arthritis can require a change in lifestyle, maybe limiting the activities you once did regularly and getting in the way of an active lifestyle.

This book will also touch on the possible causes of arthritis. Though there is some research to prove that rheumatoid arthritis can be genetic and linked to certain genes, not all arthritis types occur this way. If someone in your family like your parents or siblings have arthritis, you are more likely to have the disease too. But arthritis itself can manifest in many ways depending on the lifestyle you are living. People who have extremely physical jobs such as professional athletes or stunt performers may develop arthritis at a younger age due to the impacts on their body. Even people who perform manual labor jobs and are constantly repeating the same gestures or movements throughout their workday can have arthritis occur at those joints. Along with lifestyle, your medical history also plays a role. If you have had previous bone injuries, even with the proper treatment and healing time, it's possible that the bone and cartilage did not repair itself well. In fact, it's impossible for the repair to ever be like it was before, and any fracturing or tiny indentations can make the bone vulnerable to future breaks. People who have also battled with viral or bacterial infections, such as meningitis or staph infections, also are vulnerable due to their weakened and more fragile bones. Due to this, they may find themselves plagued with joint pain and arthritis earlier in their life.

When it comes to arthritis and inflammation, you're probably wondering what you can do to heal these aches and pains. Part of it is a natural degradation of the body, but there are many treatment options that can work to ease discomfort. Medication has advanced by leaps and bounds. Whether you're simply taking over the counter medication or stronger narcotics, it's important you first have a medical exam conducted and speak to your primary care physician about your individual care of pain. There are also individualized therapies that you can regularly attend. Whether you participate in traditional therapy, water therapy, or an exercise class, it's important that exercise and an active lifestyle becomes a part of your life, so your joints do not become even more brittle from lack of use.

This book touches on changes you can make to your diet to hopefully reduce your arthritis pain and or inflammation flare-ups. The research strongly indicates that having a balanced diet full of a variety of foods is most healthy for people battling arthritis. The more variety you consume, the more you are naturally ingesting different vitamins and minerals that your body may be lacking. Most of the time, the body processes these nutrients much better as a food item instead of over the counter vitamin supplements! Taking a pill might sound easier, but adding a vitamin or nutrient to your meals could provide you with the better benefits.

It's important to have fruits, vegetables, dairy, and grains in your diet. Each group of food provides a variety of vitamins and fiber to make your bones strong. When it comes to adjusting your diet, it's also necessary to cut out the sugary and salty processed snacks. Instead, try adding healthy snacks into your diet like beans, nuts, or yogurt. These are all proven to be very filling and may even help if you are trying to lose weight. Yogurt is even considered a superfood because it contains so many probiotics that can help your digestion! We also provide more than a dozen delicious smoothie recipes that consist of only healthy ingredients that fight against inflammation. These treats are so delicious, that you won't even remember all the health benefits associated with them! It's as simple as gathering your ingredients and pulsing your blender for a few minutes!

We hope this book is helpful to you and answers your questions on a healthy diet to reduce symptoms of arthritis and inflammation. Thank you for reading!

BONUS:

As a way of saying thank you for purchasing my book, please use your link below to claim your 3 FREE Cookbooks on Health, Fitness & Dieting Instantly

https://bit.ly/2EFv31x

You can also share your link with your friends and families whom you think that can benefit from the cookbooks or you can forward them the link as a gift!

Chapter 2: What are Arthritis and Inflammation?

If you suffer from arthritis and joint inflammation, you most likely are already familiar with the terms and key concepts behind them. For other readers, this chapter will provide an introduction into what exactly these conditions are.

Inflammation is a necessary part of the body's healing process. You may remember from high school biology that the body's white blood cells and immune system cells work in the immune system to fight off bacteria and infection for us. Inflammation occurs naturally when the body is fighting off infection. But with some diseases, the body's immune system triggers an inflammatory response even when there is no infection to fight against. These diseases are collectively called autoimmune diseases and can be very detrimental. Because the body mistakenly turns on itself and fights against normal, healthy tissue, it can greatly damage a person's system if not properly diagnosed and treated.

Arthritis is a term commonly referring to inflammation of the joints or the tissues that sound the body's joints. Arthritis itself refers to almost 200 conditions in the medical spectrum. Types of arthritis that are more commonly known are rheumatoid arthritis (RA), osteoarthritis, fibromyalgia, or lupus. Common symptoms of arthritis can involve stiffness, swelling, or pain in the joints or around the joints, but certain forms of arthritis, like lupus, can affect the body's organs and wreak havoc on the body as a whole. According to the Centers for Disease Control and Prevention (CDC), more than 50 million Americans have some form of arthritis. Although this condition is commonly associated with the elderly, it can affect people of all ages, even young children depending on what ailment they may have been diagnosed with.

Arthritis can be a range of symptoms, and it differs on how it affects an individual person in their day to day activities. Some people can experience severe pain in their joints and feel their routine is severely affected, limiting their movements and activities. Severe arthritis can make it even hard for you to lift your arms and legs. Those who have limited symptoms may be able to fight past the twinging of their knuckles or swelling they feel. There can be a decreased range of motion the more arthritis develops, along with symptoms of pain, swelling, and redness at the joints.

Rheumatoid arthritis is classified as an autoimmune disorder, or a disorder where the body turns on itself and attacks its own tissues. The body's immune system attacks the joint capsule, which is a hard membrane that covers and protects all the joints in our body. The lining becomes inflamed at the attack and a person will experience the common symptoms of swelling and pain at the joints. This disease is a complex one to diagnose because it can start so innocently with just some slight pain or swelling in the hands or wrists. We might pass it off as the usual type of aches and pains. But rheumatoid arthritis is a progressive disease. If the disease progresses without treatment, the body can even destroy the cartilage and bone within the joint. The inflammation can spread to other parts of the body and cause a severe disability. If early symptoms are noticed and seem to be getting progressively worse, a doctor will perform the necessary exams and tests to determine if and how badly the joints have been eroded. This type of arthritis seems to run in families and research has found it tied to two genetic markers. Smoking also seems to exacerbate this arthritis. Environmental factors like obesity, stressful events, and exposure to viruses or bacteria can also cause an individual to develop rheumatoid arthritis.

Juvenile idiopathic arthritis is a type of rheumatoid arthritis that affects children. According to 2015 Census data, nearly 1 in 2,000 children have this disease. If a patient has been diagnosed before the age of 16, it's counted as juvenile arthritis. Due to the young age, this disease can be even harder to identify in young adults so doctors may look at their medical history to see if they have battled any other diseases or infections. Juvenile cancer patients will tend to have this arthritis due to the weakness of their bones. Nearly 10% of juvenile arthritis patients are systemic that affect the entire body with symptoms like fever, limping, and swelling, and stiffness of the joints.

Osteoarthritis is the most common degenerative form of arthritis especially in the elderly. According to the Centers for Disease Control and Prevention, more than 30 million Americans are affected by this disease. This type of arthritis does not have inflammation as a major role in it. Neither do arthritis types such as fibromyalgia or common muscular back or neck pain. But rheumatoid arthritis, gout, and lupus are all arthritis diseases associated with inflammation in the joints. This means the inflammation of the joints does not stay localized and instead can damage other joints or the underlying bone, even turning on the body's muscles and other organs.

Although childhood arthritis is not as common, juvenile arthritis can still occur especially in children who have been exposed to bacterial or viral infections. They tend to show symptoms a lot earlier due to these infections and may have had lasting permanent damage to their joints. Sadly, there is no cure, but if caught and treated early, symptoms can be managed and contained through medication and therapy. If symptoms are noticed and do not get better, it's important a doctor do a complete medical exam to assess any damage and degradation to the joints.

Inflammation is a natural process of the body that occurs to fight diseases, infections or pathogens that are trying to attack the body. The immune system gears up for an attack on any invading cells and the body uses inflammation to fight any chemicals or irritants. Acute inflammation, or inflammation that is only temporary, is normal and a sign of a healthy body fighting back. For example, if you've cut your finger, you might feel a swelling sensation there, and the area looks red and puffy. That's a sign your body is sending cells into overdrive to heal the wound. But when the inflammation begins to occur without any infection or wound, that's a sign the body is getting mixed signals. Chronic inflammation that occurs for a long period of time can even damage internal organs if not treated. There are different inflammatory diseases that can affect the heart (myocarditis), kidneys (nephritis), eyes (iritis), and even the muscles and blood vessels (vasculitis). It can occur at multiple sites and can be tragic if caught too late. Inflammation in the lungs is very serious too and can lead to conditions like asthma and bronchitis. When the lungs become inflamed, the airways become constricted and breathing becomes more difficult. Imagine if you had just finished running a race or working out, and how you are panting for breath. With inflammation of the lungs, patients' breathing can become agitated like that without even working out or exerting themselves.

Symptoms of inflammatory arthritis do not only occur at the joints. Patients can experience other major symptoms and it's important that they are diagnosed as soon as possible. Along with pain in the joints, there could be other body pain and constant fatigue as the body tries to fight back against the inflammation. The treatments involve a combination of exercise and medication to help patients reduce the pain that is affecting their lives. Gout and lupus are two common forms of inflammatory disease. Lupus can affect so many parts of the body like the wrists, knees, and hands.

Inflammatory arthritis can be especially debilitating because it affects so many parts of the body. Along with the physical pain, a person can experience psychological stress as they cope with their symptoms and lack of body control. People in the workforce may have to leave their job due to the pain and go on disability. It's important that along with medicine and physical therapy, patients also have access to mental health resources as they adjust to the changes in their life. Often serious diseases linked to inflammation and arthritis can cause depression, mood disorders, or insomnia. A 2015 study published in JAMA Psychiatry found that patient with depression had more than 30% brain inflammation. Education on the disease and counseling from a licensed therapist are resources your doctor's office can often prescribe you. It is also beneficial to have a good support system to help with making lifestyle adjustments and keeping patients upbeat and feeling positive.

The important thing to realize about having and living with arthritis is that your entire lifestyle needs to adapt to the disease. As you are adjusting your lifestyle to cope with the pain and stiffness of your joints, you should take positive steps to maintain your activity and healthy eating habits to combat your symptoms.

Moderate exercise has been shown to be helpful in managing the pain. Losing weight might also be something your doctor recommends if you are carrying extra pounds that are putting stress on your joints. Eating a healthy diet consisting of lots of fresh fruits and vegetables is also important. This book will provide information about which foods can help combat symptoms of arthritis and inflammation. If you've successfully cut out salty or sugary snacks from your diet, we can provide you with some great ideas of what to start eating instead, like nuts and granola. Even adding some simple ingredients to your food preparation steps like ginger, garlic, turmeric powder, and using extra virgin olive oil can help you gain the beneficial properties these foods offer.

Chapter 3: The Causes of Arthritis

There are many risk factors associated with arthritis. Some types of arthritis do run in families, and you can be more likely to develop arthritis if your parents or siblings also have it. Research on rheumatoid arthritis has found it linked to genetic markers called HLA-B27 and HLA-DR4. A study of the HLA antigens in 105 unrelated American Caucasian patients with rheumatoid arthritis found that HLA-DR4 was observed in 71% cases that showed a familial trend of rheumatoid arthritis. It was also found in 63% of the non-familial cases. This correlated with another similar experiment conducted on Scandinavian patients in Finland that also found high frequencies of DR2, DR3, and DR4 in arthritis patients. These studies have allowed the scientific community to state that familial occurrence of rheumatoid arthritis could lie in these genes. If a relative has presented with the condition, then it is much more likely to show up again in the family tree.

Other types of arthritis seem to be less influenced by genetics and can be a result of other factors. Older age is the most common mark for arthritis patients because the human body's cartilage naturally becomes more brittle as we age. The older we get, the harder it is for our body to repair itself. Osteoarthritis is known as the common "wear and tear" on the body's joints and mostly occurs in individuals between 40-60 years old. Depending on other risk factors and lifestyle choices, it can even manifest itself earlier. Women are more likely than men to develop osteoarthritis though the research is not clear why that is the case. Other autoimmune diseases, like gout, tend to run higher in males.

Obesity is also a high-risk factor when it comes to developing arthritis. Those who suffer from obesity are carrying excess weight for their joints to manage, and that adds stress to the weight-bearing joints, such as the knees, spine, and hips. The extra weight greatly impacts the joints in those areas and the inflammation that occurs can gradually wear away the joint tissues. Research states that for every extra pound of weight gained, your knees gain three pounds of stress! When it comes to hips, the ratio becomes one pound of weight to six times the pressure on the hip joints! Fat tissues also can produce proteins that cause inflammation around the joints. People who have excess body fat can find themselves struggling with pain and tenderness in their joints much earlier than someone who is not obese. The cartilage at the junction of the joints begins to break down a lot earlier due to the excess weight that has become a burden to your body. That is why one of the first things a doctor will prescribe to an overweight patient exhibiting signs of arthritis is weight loss. Implementing a healthy lifestyle that promotes weight loss can sometimes help people reduce their symptoms of arthritis. They may notice a difference in their symptoms and more relief than before they had the extra pounds.

Additional risk factors to getting arthritis include previous injuries or having had infections during some point in your life. When a joint is previously broken, it can repair itself unevenly despite the injury seeming to be healed. This is especially true for sensitive areas like the wrist and the knee joint. Previous bone injuries can impact the complex structure of the bone and cartilage, so it does not react the same when faced with compression or impact. You may have heard stories of someone breaking their wrist and then many years later due to a fall or car accident, breaking it again in the same spot. This is due to the injury spot becoming more vulnerable after it was healed. It cannot hold up to a second point of impact or compression. The same is true for certain bacterial or viral infections that can affect the joint and cartilage regions. People who experience a joint infection or a staph infection have those areas of the joints deteriorated and run a higher risk for developing arthritis even after the infection has been treated. Even after the injury has healed, the cartilage repair is never the same as it once was before the injury. There could be flaws in the healing process. The damage to the joints stays and symptoms of arthritis can begin to show earlier in these patients' lives.

It's also important to understand how certain lifestyle choices can bring a higher risk of arthritis. People who tend to live a lifestyle of high sports activity or extreme physical activity can experience symptoms of arthritis earlier, such as professional athletes, stuntmen, etc. It's not only people who play contact sports, such as football or wrestling, but also sports that place repeated stress on the joints such as cycling or long distance running. The repeated activity over a period of time can break down the joints and the cartilage slowly and cause an athlete to develop arthritis even if they are not yet close to the age when arthritis usually occurs. On the reverse side, moderate exercise tends to minimize the symptoms and can actually give a muscle more strength and buoyancy. Doctors will encourage patients to implement a short exercise routine into their day to alleviate the pain and swelling in their joints. It's the repeated, long-term activity that people may be taking part in during an eight-hour a day shift at work that can cause damage. This includes even minor movements like pushing a cart or typing at a keyboard. That's often why jobs that involve manual labor or repetitive movement urge employees to stop often for breaks as a preventative measure to try and minimize damage. These employees are urged to walk around or stop their repetitive movement for at least 15 to 30 minutes every few hours to give the body a break and give those joints some relief from the repeated stress.

Despite these risk factors and environmental conditions, it's important to realize that arthritis itself is a common condition and one that scientists believe that all humans will one day afflicted with. It's only natural given the wear on our bodies and how fragile we become as we age. Whether there is a family history or not, arthritis may be a condition we all battle with in our future and one we see our elderly loved ones living with now. The next step is to educate ourselves about this disorder so we may recognize the signs and get help as needed. Whether it's medication, physical therapy, or additional supplements, your body will need help to fight this disease. Incorporating healthy eating habits into your life may be able to provide some pain relief, or at least slow the degradation of your bones as you accumulate more vitamins and minerals.

Chapter 4: Understanding Inflammation and Arthritis

In order to properly understand inflammation and the resulting joint pain, it's important to understand how the body's immune system uses inflammation in a normal way. As we discussed briefly in Chapter 1, the body's immune system composed mostly of white blood cells works to fight off infection and bacteria. It is a part of the body's healing process as cells work in overtime to fight against an infection. It's a defense system set up by our body to protect itself and white blood cells are the first line of attack. When attacked, either by an infection or an open wound of some kind, the white blood cells quickly receive growth factor hormones and send nutrients to the affected area. They swoop in and fight the infection and ingest other foreign radicals in the area. Swelling happens naturally because the movement of the blood cells and hormones to the area brings with it fluid as well. That's why the nerves at the area become so sensitive to touch.

When inflammation occurs naturally due to fighting off an infection, it's because the body releases chemicals into the bloodstream or at the affected tissues. These chemicals increase blood flow to the area and the area can turn red or warm. Sometimes the chemicals can leak fluid around the tissues and that's when swelling occurs. The nerves at the area become overstimulated and the area becomes very sensitive to touch. Have you ever noticed this when you've had an injury? The area can feel like it's burning or itching, and you can't help but feel a tingling sensation as if you want to scratch. That's because, at the localized area of the injury, cells are working together in overtime to heal you. It's the same function that occurs when you have a sore throat. The inflammation in the area is due to the body fighting against an infection. This is called acute inflammation which is simply the body reacting to a foreign agent or wound. Usually, once the infection has passed, the swelling will go away and the area will become normal again.

With inflammatory arthritis, the inflammation occurs for no reason. There is no infection or injury present that needs healing - it's simply the body turning on itself and causing the symptoms of inflammation to occur. Those symptoms such as pain, stiffness, and swelling, start affecting an individual in their daily activities and use of the joints. Eventually, the increased activity at the joints can wear down the cartilage at the bones and even cause the lining of the joints to swell. The inflammation can even begin to occur at the site of major organs, such as the eye, kidneys, lungs, or heart. Symptoms of inflammation need to be assessed immediately with a complete medical history and physical exam conducted. Other tests like X-rays and blood tests should also be studied to assess how far the damage has progressed, and if there is any way to reverse it. This type of persistent long-term inflammation is called chronic inflammation and many autoimmune disorders fall into this category. Asthma, allergies, inflammatory bowel disease, lupus, Crohn's disease... all these fall in the category of diseases with chronic inflammation. The body mistakenly sends signals to the organs to become inflamed even though there is no threat. The white blood cells arrive at the area and find no threat, so they begin attacking the body's own cells and tissues.

It's hard to imagine the scientific phenomenon of pain, but the sensation of pain is the body's response to warn us regarding an injury. In the case of arthritis, there is an injury to your joints which the body is becoming aware of and is sending out alert signals about. The damaged tissue around the joints releases neurotransmitter chemicals that carry the message up your spinal cord and to your brain. The brain processes the signal it received and sends a signal back to your motor nerves to respond. For example, when you cut yourself, the message is instantly sent to your brain and you move your hand away.

It's important to note that the commonly known ailments of muscle pain and back pain are not necessarily tied to arthritis and joint pain. Soft tissue pain is felt in the tissues rather than the joints. It tends to occur when parts of the body are overused repeatedly, or due to an injury. Back pain can be due to many factors, such as damage to the nerves, bones, joints, muscles, or ligaments. If these symptoms are temporary and can be relived easily enough with medication or a massage, they would not fall under the category of chronic inflammation which continues to occur for a longer period of time.

Chapter 5: How to Manage Arthritis Pain

The good news is that science has progressed rapidly to battle the types of arthritis discovered. These diseases are often diagnosed correctly now instead of simply passed off as "creaky old bones", especially in elderly patients. Non-inflammatory types of arthritis can often be treated with over the counter pain medications. Often a lifestyle change, such as weight loss, and a routine of physical activity can help to relieve symptoms.

In fact, doctors will often prescribe physical therapy to help elderly or sedentary arthritis patients become gradually more familiar with physical activity. This is especially true for elderly patients who are finding it hard to be mobile and need a push to incorporate an exercise regime into their lifestyle. Individual physical therapy is geared specifically for what the patient needs and what is the best remedy for their condition. Whether it's arm joint pain or knee pain, your therapist would work with you to create a routine to exercise the affected joint area. Sometimes a therapist may also use massage techniques, or use ice or heat packs to relieve pain.

Water therapy is also a great form of specialized therapy that can provide ease for patients. Water supports an individual's weight and puts less pressure on the muscles and joints. It provides resistance to your muscles which in turn exercises them and makes them stronger. This is very helpful for patients who might be overweight and just beginning to exercise. It gives a person, especially an older person, a buoyancy and lightness to help them feel more agile than they may have in years! Many people mistakenly think of aquatic exercises as swimming or diving, but that's not the case.

Instead, these are simply exercises that are performed while the person is standing in water that is about waist or shoulder level. Regularly performing aquatic exercises can help relieve pain in patients and improve the movement in their hip or knee joints.

Therapy can be something you pay for or is prescribed by your doctor if you need more specialized care, but regular old fashioned exercise is something any doctor will recommend. (Keep in mind, this varies case to case because someone's arthritis may be more severe or coupled with other illnesses.) Exercise is considered one of the best ways to manage pain in osteoarthritis patients. Their pain can even be reduced if they regularly exercise. Walking is one of the best ways to exercise without adding too much stress on the joints. As an aerobic exercise, it also strengthens the heart and lowers blood pressure. In arthritis patients specifically, it tones the muscles that support joints in the body, and as you age, it can slow the loss of bone mass. Studies have found that people who have arthritis but who participated faithfully in an exercise routine were less likely to need hip replacement surgery compared to arthritis patients who did not exercise. The patients who exercised even reported having overall better physical health and more flexibility and range of motion.

There are a few types of exercises that are recommended for arthritis patients to help ease their pain and the stiffness in their motions.

- Flexibility exercises: These exercises refer to the range of motion a patient may be having difficulty with. For example, the joint is not moving to the full motion that it used to before. Maybe someone is having knee pain where they cannot stretch their leg as they used to before. Flexibility exercises focus on gently stretching and expanding the range of movement at that joint. A therapist may first show you what type of exercises to perform and how to stretch the joint and the surrounding muscles, but these exercises can easily be performed in the comfort of your home without help. Performing them regularly can help flexibility return in those joints. It's like the old saying goes - practice makes perfect! You may not get back complete range of motion, but it may certainly be better than before.

- Strengthening exercises: These exercises work to strengthen the muscles. Strong muscles work to protect the joints in the body. The stronger your muscles are, the more cushion they can provide joints that are affected by arthritis. Strengthening exercises can be done with a medium to light range of weights, and ones that can be attached to your feet to strengthen leg muscles. These exercises should also be done many times a week to continue to exercise the muscles and build endurance.

- Endurance exercises: These are also called aerobic exercises because they strengthen the heart muscle. These exercises include things like walking, bicycling, swimming, or using the elliptical or treadmill machine. Activities like this build up a person's stamina and make their lungs more efficient. Not only that, but it also provides physical exercise for the whole body, allowing you to stretch and exercise many joints, muscles, and ligaments.

When it comes to deciding how often you should exercise, it's important that each patient follow their physical therapist or doctor's advice. Generally, flexibility or range-of-motion exercises should be done every day to help the joint become familiar with the new stretches. Other exercises should be done for a minimum of 20 minutes a few times a week, but it all depends on how vigorous the exercise is performed. It's also important that patients be aware of their own arthritis and the fragility of their condition. Depending on age, the severity of the disease, and range of motion, your activities should fit your abilities and your lifestyle. For example, someone elderly with severe arthritis should be playing a high impact sport, but stay limited to their flexibility exercises. Someone younger may still be able to jog or swim a few times a week to keep their joints and muscles strong and their heart healthy. Arthritis patients will want to be move slowly and carefully in their routine as to avoid any fractures or injuries. Always be sure to warm up and cool down with enough stretching time before and after working out to properly relax your muscles!

There are many categories of medication that also assist with joint pain and inflammation. There are non-steroidal anti-inflammatory drugs that reduce pain and inflammation. These tend to be available over the counter, such as Advil, Motrin, and Aleve. They are even available as creams or patches to be applied to the problem area for ease. This is great for traveling, or to have applied if you will be sitting for a long period of time. Analgesics is a category or medication that can reduce the pain of arthritis but will not affect inflammation. Tylenol, or acetaminophen, is available over the counter, but narcotics like Percocet, Oxycontin, or Vicodin can only be prescribed by a doctor. Before a patient progresses to stronger drugs that contain oxycodone or hydrocodone, he or she would need to have battled arthritis for a longer period of time and not found relief with alternative methods. Because these drugs have addictive properties, their use would need to be carefully monitored by a doctor.

For arthritis associated with inflammation, disease-modifying antirheumatic drugs work to stop the immune system from attacking itself and the joints, or at least slow down the attack. These medications are prescribed to rheumatoid arthritis patients. Corticosteroids suppress the immune system and work to reduce inflammation at the sight of the pain. Patients with more serious inflammation disorders that are classified as autoimmune disorders would need to be monitored carefully with regular testing and doctor's visits.

As we mentioned in the previous chapter, obesity is also a risk factor for arthritis. Because of this, it makes sense that one of the first things that a doctor would prescribe to an obese patient is weight loss. The more excess body weight you are carrying, the faster the progression of arthritis can occur as well. The cartilage at the joints begins to wear down faster as a result of the excess weight it has been carrying. Losing weight can reduce the stress on the joints. People will often notice an ease in their arthritis symptoms when they lose a significant amount of weight and maintain a lifestyle that keeps the pounds off. They begin to feel better physically and experience a wider range of motion than they did before. This is simply to state that a patient should not be offended if they are recommended to lose weight by a doctor. The research shows that it will be beneficial in the long run.

Chapter 6: Healthy Eating Habits

To follow a routine of eating healthy to combat your arthritis, it's important to be aware of what kind of diet you need to set. You should be sure to eat nutrient-rich foods and avoid sugary or fatty snacks that can cause inflammation or trigger weight gain that would further exacerbate your arthritis. Research suggests that the type of diet you are eating, coupled with whether you are exercising, can play a major factor in the progression of your disease and the symptoms you exhibit. There is no magic cure for these diseases, but a variety of foods and a balanced diet can benefit a person who has symptoms of arthritis.

Research regarding patients and dairy ingredients have come up inconclusive despite evidence showing both sides. A 2015 study in the Journal of Nutrition found that eating dairy foods increased inflammation in a group of adults selected for the sample. A similar study found that osteoarthritis patients who ate more dairy were more likely to need surgery for a hip replacement. On the other hand, numerous studies show that eating more yogurt and drinking more milk can lower the risk of gout, an autoimmune disease we mentioned earlier that also showcases arthritis. The conflicting evidence can leave patients torn about how to incorporate dairy into their daily diet.

Most research has painted dairy products in a positive picture. A recent 2017 study found that dairy does have beneficial anti-inflammatory effects except for in people who are allergic to cow's milk. Keep in mind that "dairy" does not just refer to milk, but also ice cream, cheese, and yogurt. There are many food items to consider in that category. The good news is that research on yogurt has come back consistently positive. The probiotics in it are associated with decreased insulin resistance and decreased inflammation in the body. Just like with any other diet, moderation is key. Overeating high-fat dairy products or sweetened products will not help in terms of weight loss which is also very important to minimize inflammation.

Some people find that avoiding certain foods can reduce their arthritic flare-ups. For example, if a certain type of milk is associated with negative symptoms, you can try an elimination diet and quit eating it for a while. This can show you how your body responds, and it's possible you feel better without cow's milk.

Another debate that has sprung up is the concept of organic foods. There is no strong evidence that supports eating organic food can minimize your chances of getting autoimmune diseases or arthritis. But it can make sense to minimize your exposure to unwanted chemicals by choosing an organic diet. When you eat foods that are from conventional farms that use hormones or chemicals, you're ingesting that as well every time you have eggs, meat, or cheese. But besides that, logical fallacy, there's no evidence that states conventional food is bad for people with arthritis. It's important that even if you are not buying organic produce, you still are consuming a diet full of a variety of fruits and vegetables. All fruits and vegetables should be washed thoroughly or in a water and vinegar rinse to remove any harmful pesticide residues. If you can afford it, try buying some organic produce, like the ones with soft exterior skins that you directly consume such as peaches, spinach, or bell peppers. The consensus by doctors has been that a serving of at least 5 fruits and vegetables a day is considered healthy for an arthritis patient. If you are concerned about possible pesticides or growth hormones, buying organic or non-GMO foods is a personal choice up to you.

Antioxidants in produce tend to fight inflammation and are also a major source of nutrients. Having a variety of fruits and vegetables gives you the ability to take in more vitamins and nutrients. Try to incorporate vegetables into your snacks more. For example, if you're having a sandwich, instead of just a slice of cheese or some low-sodium meat slices, add in some vegetables so you're getting a serving of produce as well. If you're planning on having a salad, try adding in some fruit or nuts to increase the proteins you're taking in, and surprise your taste buds!

When it comes to meat and seafood choices in your diet, fish is encouraged as it provides a great source of anti-inflammatory omega-3 fatty acids. It can be substituted easily for red meat in your diet, especially if you are at risk for high disease or have high cholesterol. If you are not familiar with where to start when it comes to choosing fish, there are dozens of varieties for you to choose from! If your local grocery store does not have many options, try finding a local fish market to find fresh options. Avoid processed meats that tend to contain preservatives and are high in sodium. Try to buy more lean cuts of meat with fat trimmed off. Turkey and chicken are also healthier substitutes to red meat.

Make room in your diet for whole grains like cereal and pasta. Instead of white rice that tends to be high in carbohydrates, try experimenting with alternatives like quinoa or wheat. You can even find pasta that are made of vegetables or chickpeas so that they are lower in starches and sugars. Be sure to read the ingredients when trying new items to be sure you are getting the protein you need, and that items are low in sugar and carbohydrates.

Try and cut out packaged and processed snacks from your diet. The sugar and salt content in these products cause health concerns and are not helpful to a weight loss lifestyle. There are healthier alternatives out there that have their snacks based on vegetable or legumes instead, like lentil chips or roasted garbanzo beans. Be sure to read the label carefully when finding a new snack to make sure it's as healthy as it could be addictive! If your local grocery store does not have many healthy options, you may have to find a local organic grocery store or browse online to see what options are available. This also includes being careful of what canned foods you buy. You want to be sure you always drain the liquid in the cans and rinse the beans, or fruit, or whatever you are going to be eating. You want to be sure the fruits have preserved in their own juice, not in a sugary syrup that packs on calories. There are tons of canned beans and lentils out there that are easy to store and make to whip up a quick vegetarian recipe. Be sure that the sodium level is 5% or less per serving.

It's important to note that there is no research that proves abiding by a vegan or vegetarian diet could be the cure to inflammation. In fact, studies on this have been mixed. Some studies found that people who were strictly on a vegetarian diet had no alleviation of pain or stiffness in their joints compared to the control group that followed a traditional diet with meat. Other studies have found that patients who followed a vegan diet for months at a time tended to have improvement in their swollen joints and less stiffness in the morning compared to the control group. With these mixed results, doctors will not urge you to follow a vegan or vegetarian lifestyle. It is important to note though that a meat-free lifestyle can lead to lower cholesterol and blood pressure levels and decrease your chances of becoming obese. But there are also downsides to these diet choices. Vegetarians, and especially vegans, tend to have lower levels of vitamins in their blood, as well as low calcium and fatty acids. These substances are crucial to bone health. Vegetarians also tend to have lower levels of HDL which is the "good cholesterol".

If you are considering making a major change in your diet plan to help with your inflammation or arthritis, it's important you first speak to your doctor about the risks and reasons. There are other ways you can reduce your meat intake such as adding a "Meatless Monday" to your weekly schedule or incorporating a side of vegetables or a salad more often. If you do decide to cut meat entirely from your diet, then your doctor may need to run a blood test to see if there are any vitamin supplements you should be taking orally.

Foods That Fight Arthritis

Although there is no direct cure for arthritis and it is really a balanced lifestyle of exercise, diet, and medication, some foods are believed to fight arthritis. Adding these items to your regular diet could ease your symptoms of inflammation. Here is a beginners list to what you should try and incorporate into your meals!

- **Fish**: Fish is a source of high protein and packed with omega-3 fatty acids that fight inflammation. Doctors recommend at least 3 to 4 ounces of fish consumed twice a week. Tuna, mackerel, herring, salmon... whatever your favorite is, try having it for dinner once or twice a week to get the nutrients you need.

- **Tofu**: If you're a vegetarian and do not have fish or meat as a protein source, soybeans such as tofu and edamame are great alternatives that can also provide omega-3 fatty acids. These substitutes are high in protein but low in fat which makes them a great substitute.

- **Extra virgin olive oil**: This oil was considered a luxury in the past because it has medicinal properties similar to anti-inflammatory drugs. When battling arthritis, it's important to even be aware of the type of cooking oil we are using. Including olive oil, walnut oil, safflower oil, and avocado oil also have properties that can lower cholesterol and a high content of omega-3 fatty acids.

- **Berries**: Anthocyanins have been researched and found to have an anti-inflammatory effect and can reduce the frequency of gout attacks in patients with that autoimmune disorder. Along with these health benefits, anthocyanins tend to give fruits their rich purple or red color, like in cherries, strawberries, blueberries, and blackberries. The whole berry family!

- **Dairy**: Despite what we mentioned earlier about the studies conducted on dairy and arthritis symptoms, milk, cheese, and yogurt are all packed with Vitamin D and calcium which are essential for the body. They are both necessary to increase bone strength, so it's important they be consumed on a moderate basis. If you are lactose intolerant or have a dairy sensitivity, then you will have to search for substitutes that work for you. Leafy vegetables and lentils are a great substitute for those who may be allergic to dairy.

- **Garlic**: Studies have found that people who ate more foods from the allium family, like onions, leeks, and garlic, showed fewer signs of osteoarthritis. Raw garlic itself is found to have many health benefits like lowering blood sugar levels and regulating blood pressure. You want to try and consume it in its raw or semi-cooked form as much as you can though because it loses many of those properties once cooked. Garlic has been found to even block the presence of enzymes that damage cartilage in the body - which is great news for arthritis patients. So, mince some raw garlic and add it as a garnish on your soup or salad to gain the benefits it can provide!

- **Broccoli:** Broccoli is rich in vitamins C and K, and contains a compound called sulforaphane which researchers believe can slow the progress of osteoarthritis. It is also rich in calcium which is beneficial for building strong bones.

- **Green tea**: We've been hearing for years about the benefits of this drink and the antioxidants it provides the body. Researchers have studied the antioxidant epigallocatechin-3-gallate (EGCG) that stops the production of molecules that causes joint damage in patients with rheumatoid arthritis. If you've been an avid coffee drinker, try a cup of green tea instead!

- **Citrus:** Grapefruits, oranges, clementines... you name it! The citrus family is rich in vitamins and that works to prevent arthritis and maintain healthy joints in the body. Another great tip is to use fresh lemon or lime juice in recipes instead of the concentrated kind.

- **Nuts**: Nuts are one of those rare treats that are high in good fats, so they are considered "heart healthy", in moderation, of course. They also contain many beneficial vitamins like calcium, zinc, vitamin E, protein, and fiber. They are helpful if you are trying to lose weight because a handful of them can be very filling and allow you to cut back on the portions you're consuming. There are tons of options out there for you to find exactly which is the perfect nut for you. Pistachios, almonds, walnuts, pine nuts, macadamia nuts... it's all out there! Be sure that you are consuming these nuts in their raw form though. If you are leaning more toward the chocolate covered or salted version then you are canceling out the health benefits.

- **Whole Grains**: While most diets would urge you to stay away from carbohydrates, whole grains are unique because they provide the beneficial effect of lowering the levels of C-reactive protein in the blood. C-reactive protein tends to be found with signs of inflammation in the body and is associated with an increased risk of diabetes, rheumatoid arthritis, and even heart disease. Including things like rice, whole-grain cereals, and low-fat oatmeal in your diet is a terrific way to maintain low levels of this protein in your bloodstream. Research has shown that people who had fewer servings of whole grains in their diet tended to have higher inflammation markers. The fiber found in whole grains also helps with weight loss.

- **Beans**: Beans a great and inexpensive source of healthy vitamins and minerals such as zinc, potassium, iron, and protein. Beans and legumes are well known for the benefits they provide to the immune system. You don't have to create a fancy recipe if you don't know how to incorporate them into a meal - just have canned beans handy and add a handful to your salad or rice bowl. Kidney beans, pinto beans, and red beans are especially great to keep the heart healthy.

Foods That Fight Inflammation

As stated above, there is no direct cure for arthritis and it is all about managing a healthy lifestyle that includes your diet, exercise, and medication if needed. Researchers have found that a diet resembling a Mediterranean diet is actually very helpful to fight inflammation. This diet is comprised of lots of vegetables, fish, and using olive oil instead of a different type of oil in cooking. There are some foods that have proven to be beneficial and can combat symptoms of arthritis. Adding these to your regular diet could ease your symptoms. Here is a beginners list to what you should try and shop for and incorporate into your meals!

- **Fish**: As stated above, fish is a great alternative to red meat, especially in patients who are also battling high cholesterol or at risk of heart disease. Fish contains high amounts of omega-3 fatty acids that work to reduce the amounts of interleukin-6 and C-reactive protein (CPR) in the body. These two proteins are involved in creating inflammation in the body. Research encourages inflammation patients to have at least 3 to 4 ounces of fish twice a week. Whether it's tuna, sardines, salmon, herring, or mackerel... pick a type of fish that you enjoy the most and give it a place in your weekly menu. Grilled, smoked, fried... the options are endless!

- **Colorful Fruits**: Anthocyanins are antioxidants found naturally in colorful fruit such as raspberries, blackberries, cherries, and strawberries. It's also found in high amounts in leafy vegetables like broccoli, kale, and spinach. These work to naturally fight inflammation in the body. Be sure to incorporate at least 2 to 3 servings of fruits and vegetables in your day. It's all about having a variety of those fruits so you can naturally take in as many antioxidants as you can. Watermelon is especially beneficial because it contains choline, an inhibitor that blocks signs of inflammation in the body's white blood cell network.

- **Nuts or Seeds**: Nuts are great snack items that are full of monosaturated fat, or the "good fat" that works to fight inflammation in the body. On top of that, they're full of fiber and very filling. They're a great addition to your diet, especially if you're trying to cut back on how much you are eating throughout the day. This can work to fill you up, fight inflammation, and may even help you lose a few pounds! There are tons of healthy options for nuts so browse the snack aisle and see which your favorites are. There's walnuts, pistachios, almonds, or a healthy trail mix combination of all the above! Be sure that you are picking natural nuts without any additives or sugar or salt which would defeat the purpose of such a healthy snack. Try and eat a handful of nuts a day to fight inflammation and increase your "good" cholesterol levels.

- **Beans:** Beans are another substance that naturally have anti-inflammation compounds and are packed with antioxidants. And they're very cost efficient too! You can buy them already prepared in cans or buy a big bag to keep in your pantry. They are packed with lots of nutrients like folic acid, protein, iron, potassium, and zinc too. There are also many varieties out there so you can pick and choose which you prefer.

Black beans, pinto beans, garbanzo beans, red kidney beans... we hope you have a favorite that you can incorporate into your diet at least twice a week.

- **Olive Oil**: There's a reason olive oil is sometimes referred to as "nectar of the gods". It contains heart-healthy monosaturated fats and tons of natural antioxidants that work to lower inflammation in the body. Just a few teaspoons used in cooking can be enough for you to gain the benefits of this miraculous oil. Extra virgin olive oil is less processed and contains even more nutrients than standard olive oil. It can be on the pricey side though, so you can save it for use on salads as a dressing or in soups. You want to be sure that when ingesting olive oil you are keeping it at low or room temperature. High heat destroys the structure of the polyphenols in the oil or the natural compounds that elicit the health benefits we described. Avoid using it for frying or baking, but be sure to incorporate it into your salad dressings or adding a little to your pasta before a meal.

- **Fiber**: Fiber is another excellent source that works to reduce inflammation in the body. It lowers the amount of C-reactive proteins (CPR) in the bloodstream (these are one of many proteins that cause inflammation). Research has found that ingesting fiber through food works better to lower CPR levels than simply taking over the counter supplements. Because of this, it's important that patients have a fiber-rich diet. Whether it's coming from vegetables (like potatoes, celery, or carrots), fruits (bananas, apples, and oranges) or from whole grains (like oatmeal or fiber-rich cereal), be sure you have a fiber-rich diet. You can also ask your doctor about adding a fiber supplement to your diet if you feel you aren't eating enough.

- **Onions**: Leeks, onions, garlic, and green onions... all these members of the allium family are linked to lowering inflammation in the body. Onions contain quercetin, a compound that inhibits histamines that cause inflammation, like when you have an allergy attack and your lungs become inflamed. They are packed with beneficial antioxidants and have many health benefits. Not only do they reduce inflammation, but also reduce the risk of heart disease and lower levels of LDL which is the "bad" cholesterol in the body. Try and incorporate onions into your meals, whether it's dicing them and adding them into your vegetables, grilling them with your meat, or including them in your pasta or sandwiches. If you don't like raw onions, you can always sauté them with a little seasoning - but go light on the salt and oil!

- **Drink Moderately**: Resveratrol, a compound found in red wine, is believed to have anti-inflammatory effects. So, sure, maybe a glass of red wine every now and again can have medicinal effects. But it is important to remember that people with rheumatoid arthritis should limit their alcohol intake, especially with higher dose medications. If you are a drinker, be sure to have a talk with your doctor about how much you are drinking and if it's okay with the medication you are taking.

- **Avoid Processed Foods**: We all know potato chips and other snacks in the junk food aisle are delicious, but the truth is, these snacks are not helping you gain any relief from inflammation. In fact, the additional salt in chips and other snacks can cause inflammation in the bloodstream as your body struggles to process the increase in sodium. In fact, a study at Yale University in 2013 showed an increased risk of having rheumatoid arthritis if they were more prone to a salty diet. This study has yet to be confirmed with more research but any doctor can confirm that extra salt is not a good thing for the body. An increase in processed foods can lead to weight gain which can increase your symptoms as your body adjusts to the more pounds you're carrying. Gaining a few pounds might not sound drastic to you, but the body's joints have to overcompensate for the new weight. Avoid these processed foods and try and stick with healthy snacks like nuts and whole grain granola for snacking.

Foods that Boost the Immune System

If you're looking into items that work to boost your immune system, here are some foods that researchers have found to have healthy benefits! It always helps to bolster your immune system and give you a better chance of fighting off infections. Though there are plenty of over the counter supplements, here are some items you can add to your diet to give you the same benefits.

- **Citrus Fruits:** Extensive research has shown that this family of fruits is loaded with high amounts of Vitamin C. This is especially necessary for the immune system because Vitamin C is believed to increase white blood cell production. White blood cells? Well, those are the first "soldiers" in the line of defense of your immune system to protect you against infections. Popular citrus fruits include grapefruits, oranges, tangerines, and clementines. Also, don't forget to use natural and organic lime and lemon juice whenever you can and in your cooking, as opposed to the ones from concentrate.

- **Bell Peppers**: Here's a fun fact - one ounce of bell pepper contains two times as much vitamin C as an ounce of fruit from the citrus family! Something about the color that gives this pepper its red quality also provides it with a stunning amount of vitamin C. These peppers also are packed with beta-carotene which keeps your skin and eyes healthy. With a beautiful selection of colors available, these are great to add to your salad or slaws. They add some color to your food and give you great health benefits too!

- **Yogurt:** Yogurt is a natural source of probiotics or "good" bacteria that live in your gut and help to digest foods. Not only that, but it also works to boost immunity. You want to be sure that you are avoiding heavily sweetened yogurts though because those tend to cancel out the positive health benefits. Try to find yogurts with fewer additives and be wary of ones that come packed with fruit. You can always add in your own fruit or granola to be sure you are getting all the health benefits!

- **Ginger**: Ginger is found to reduce inflammation and is perfect to reduce a sore throat or swollen glands if you are fighting off a cold. Just imagine having a hot cup of ginger tea when you're home sick with a fever! It's also been found to reduce nausea and lower cholesterol. If you are not able to eat a piece of ginger raw, have a mincer or zester handy so you can at least sprinkle some over your pasta or salads. Researchers at the University of Wisconsin found a few other spices that also have anti-inflammatory properties – oregano, cloves, nutmeg, and rosemary. If you're already a big spice lover, try and incorporate more of these into your recipes. If you're a newbie simply trying to gain the health benefits, experiment with these new flavors in your meals. You may find something delicious and healthy too!

- **Chicken or Turkey**: Along with all the other health benefits of white meat over red meat, chicken and turkey also contain high amounts of B-6 vitamins. Just 3 ounces of white meat contains nearly half your daily recommended amount! This vitamin is a very important part of the chemical reactions that occur in the immune system to form new red blood cells and keep them healthy. Chicken stock or soup that's made from boiling chicken bones also contains nutrients that help with immunity. There's a reason why they say chicken soup is the best medicine!

- **Shellfish**: Zinc is an important mineral that our body needs to instruct our immune cells how to function and which infections to fight. It's also very important in healing open wounds! Shellfish is a category of seafood that includes lobster, clams, mussels, and crab. Keep in mind that you want to have shellfish in moderate doses. Too much zinc in the bloodstream can inhibit the function of the immune system. Men should have about 11 milligrams a day, and women should have 8 milligrams.

- **Tea**: A Harvard study found that participants who drank at least 5 cups of black tea a day had nearly 10 times more interferons (proteins that signal amongst each other to fight viruses) in their bloodstream than participants who drank a placebo drink. L-theanine is an amino acid that is present in black and green tea. If you're already an avid tea drinker, try and stick to these types of tea. Be sure to get out all the nutrients you can from the tea bag before tossing it out!

- **Garlic**: Garlic naturally contains the ingredient of allicin which works to fight infections and bacteria in the body's immune system. A study in Great Britain found that out of 146 people given either garlic or a placebo for a period of 12 weeks, the ones given garlic were two-thirds less likely to catch a cold. Try and incorporate a clove or two of garlic in your meals, even if you're mincing it and adding it on top as a garnish.

- **Eggs**: We already know that eggs are a major source of protein, but they also are necessary for a healthy immune system. Eggs are rich in Vitamin D that is important for your bones. A deficiency in Vitamin D can increase your chances of upper respiratory infections during the winter, and even immune disorders like diabetes. Immune cells even have cell receptors that are constantly searching for vitamin D in the bloodstream! While you can get vitamin D through sun exposure as well, it's important that you are eating plenty of foods high in Vitamin D such as fish, beef, and eggs so that you are including it in your diet even in the winter season. Try and switch to a Vitamin D fortified milk too!

- **Fish**: We've been saying it repeatedly, but it's the truth - fish is packed with tons of omega-3 fatty acids that work to strengthen the immune system and potentially ease symptoms of arthritis and inflammation. Research has found that these fatty acids can fortify the lungs from a cold, reduce inflammation, and even protect you from the flu. Whatever type of fish you prefer (and there are tons out there to choose from!), be sure to have fish as a meal at least twice a week. For high cholesterol and heart disease patients, it's also a great alternative to red meat.

Vegetables to Include in Your Diet

If you're focusing more on which vegetables to shop for, here are some great suggestions that are full of beneficial vitamins and minerals. They might even help you strengthen your immune system if you are already fighting an illness, or simply trying not to get a cold this winter!

- **Broccoli**: We've heard it from childhood and that's because it's the truth - broccoli is good for your immune system. It has vitamins A, E, C, fiber, and natural antioxidants that work to strengthen the immune system. It contains high amounts of sulforaphane, an antioxidant that fights to reduce levels of NF-kB in your bloodstream. NF-kB is responsible for inflammation flare-ups in the body. The key to getting the most health benefits from broccoli is to cook it as little as possible. If you can eat it raw - even better! If not, lightly sauté it with a minimum amount of oil and seasoning. Other cruciferous vegetables that are associated with anti-inflammatory benefits include Brussels sprouts, cabbage, and cauliflower.

- **Sweet Potatoes**: Instead of the regular brown skin potatoes, sweet potato actually contains more beta-carotene which your body metabolizes into vitamin A that helps the immune system. Beta-carotene rich foods are identified easily by their bright orange pigment - sweet potatoes, carrots, squash, and cantaloupe. All are great sources to help your body intake vitamin A to help your immune system. A great way to enjoy your sweet potato is to load them with other healthy foods like a dollop of sour cream, a sprinkle of turmeric spice, herbs, and lemon or lime juice.

- **Spinach**: Another vegetable that haunts some us from our childhood dinner table, spinach is packed with lots of Vitamin C, and other antioxidants that help the immune system fight off infections. Like broccoli, the more raw you can consume it, the more health benefits you will gain. If you can have it added raw in your salad, that's the best option. But you can also sauté it lightly and have as a vegetable side.

- **Mushrooms**: The benefits of mushrooms have become more well-known in the last few decades and it's a well-deserved honor they're getting at the salad bar. Numerous studies show that mushrooms increase the production of white blood cells which is very helpful if you are sick or fighting a disease or infection. Reishi, maitake, shiitake mushrooms, and Portobello mushrooms have been found to help bolster immunity the most. Mushrooms are low in calories but high in vitamins, lectins, and phenols - all of which work together to fight against inflammation in the body. Whether it's on your pizza, sautéed as a side, or added to your pasta, be sure to include mushrooms in your diet when you can to get the benefits they offer. The less cooked you can eat them, the better it is for you to gain their full anti-inflammatory effect.

- **Kale**: There's a reason this vegetable is everywhere these days! Kale is a great source of vitamin A which works to strengthen your immune system in fighting off infections. Whether it's in a salad or a smoothie, or just added on as an afterthought in your pasta, try and incorporate a few servings of this in your diet throughout the week to get your recommended vitamin A intake. Like spinach that we mentioned above, leafy green vegetables like kale are a great source of anti-inflammatory agents. So whether you prefer spinach, kale, Swiss chard, or arugula, be sure to incorporate some of these greens into your diet!

- **Tomatoes**: Tomatoes contain high amounts of lycopene. Lycopene has been found to reduce the amount of inflammatory proteins in the bloodstream. A 2014 study even found that women who drank tomato juice regularly decreased their inflammation flare-ups. More helpful than taking lycopene supplements, ingesting raw tomatoes and tomato products are more helpful to reduce inflammation. It's important to note that lycopene is a fat-soluble nutrient, which means it's absorbed better by the body when it's paired with some fat at the same time. So, tomatoes are great to pair with some cheesy pasta, or added as a topping to your pizza!

- **Beets**: The rich red color of beets is due to high amounts of phytonutrients that the vegetable contains. Beets have high amounts of minerals and vitamins and contain the amino acid betaine. Betaine is found to help the liver function, detoxify cells from any toxins in the environment, and help cells maintain their health and normal function in the immune system. They've even been found to protect the body against heart disease and cancer, and are considered a "brain food", or a food that helps increase blood flow to the brain. Try and incorporate beets into your salads and include it in your vegetable drawer.

- **Soy**: Tofu, edamame, and soy milk are all great ways to absorb the healthy benefits of soy products. Isoflavones that are present in soy products can be linked to lower inflammation in patients, and women specifically. Soy also helps keep the bones and heart healthy. Try and use soy milk when making smoothies so you can enjoy the benefits of it coupled with all the other fruits and veggies you are eating.

Shopping Guide

So what tips can we give you to plan for a better diet that can hopefully reduce the symptoms of arthritis and inflammation in your life? It's important that you know what foods you should be stocking up in your pantry, and what types of food you should be avoiding altogether. Here are some tips to get you started when you're browsing the grocery store aisles!

- **Fresh Fruits and Vegetables**: We've seen with the many examples listed above that a wide variety of fruits and vegetables consumed allow you to intake the most vitamins and minerals in your diet. Try and find fresh produce. If you cannot afford organic produce, that's okay, but try and buy a few things organic such as leafy green vegetables like kale and spinach, or soft-flesh fruits where the skin will be eaten, like peaches and plums. Different colored fruits also have different beneficial properties, like red fruits and vegetables (apples, red bell peppers, strawberries), as well as darker skin fruits and vegetables (blackberries, eggplants, blueberries), so be sure to have a colorful array of items in your shopping cart!

- **Chicken and Turkey:** These poultry items are great alternatives to red meat, especially for patients who might already be battling high cholesterol or heart disease. Try and find fresh cuts and avoid processed or pre-made frozen meals that could have preservatives or high amounts of sodium.

- **Fish**: The benefits of omega-3 fatty acids have been praised over and over in this chapter, so we urge you to buy some fish this grocery trip! Whether it's tuna, mackerel, salmon, or tilapia, explore your options and recipes so you can incorporate fish into your meals at least twice a week.

- **Olive Oil**: The benefits of olive oil are like ibuprofen, but naturally! It's found to lower inflammation and reduce pain. Be sure that you have olive oil to use when cooking or as dressing on salads and pasta. Try and find brands that come with a seal of approval like the North American Olive Oil Seal. If you can splurge on extra virgin olive oil which is less refined, even better! But regular olive oil should become a staple in your pantry.

- **Whole Wheat Grains and Cereals:** Try and find grains that are whole wheat without any sodium or additives. Also look for cereals that are packed with iron or fiber, so you are hitting your daily intake limit without needing to take over the counter supplements.

- **Yogurt and Dairy**: Despite some studies that have dairy as aggravating arthritis symptoms, yogurts, milk, and cheeses provide many health benefits.

- **Ginger and Garlic:** As stated above, ginger and garlic are two substances that have natural ingredients that reduce inflammation in the body. Try and incorporate these two foods in your diet whether it's minced garlic on a salad or crushed ginger in soups or slaws.

- **Juices:** As mentioned above, many vegetable juices have been linked to decreased inflammation such as tomato juice and beet juice. It's important that these juices contain fewer sugars and additives. They should use the most organic ingredients possible. Whether you're making them at home or finding them at the grocery store, be sure that you are keeping the fruit or vegetable in as pure a state as you can.

- **Teas**: Herbal green tea has been found to have antioxidant and anti-inflammatory properties. A study at Washington State University found that a molecule in green tea works to target a pro-inflammatory protein that is found in high quantities in patients with rheumatoid arthritis. It is important to note that green tea contains traces of vitamin K which can counteract blood thinners. If you are on blood thinners, it's important you talk to your doctor before you incorporate green tea into your diet.

- Avoid Processed Sugary Foods: Sorry, but junk food has to stay in the store! If you are trying to maintain a healthy lifestyle and promote weight loss, stay away from processed snacks that are loaded with sugars or corn syrup. Try and find alternatives that fall under "healthy snacking" such as lentil chips or salt-free popcorn.

Chapter 7: Drinks & Smoothies That Reduce Inflammation

As discussed in the previous chapter, many foods, especially fruits and vegetables, can fight symptoms of inflammation and arthritis. It's all about adjusting your diet to a healthy one full of lots of good fats and a variety of vitamins and minerals. You also want to make sure you're avoiding trans fats, alcohol, and sugars that can cause flare-ups of inflammation. You want to increase foods in your diet that agree with your digestion and that are helpful to fight inflammation.

Smoothies are a great way to pack a lot of vitamins and minerals into just one cup. They're easy to make and easy to take on the go! Gathering the right ingredients is simple as long as you have them already stocked in your fridge and pantry. That's where the helpful shopping guide in the earlier chapter comes handy! To make it even easier on yourself amid a busy schedule, you can even portion out ingredients and keep them in freezer-safe bags so it's as easy as pouring and mixing your smoothie.

You want to pack your drinks with many of the ingredients we mentioned that can combat signs of inflammation. Here are some additions that go well in smoothies to further help you and your health.

✓ **Turmeric**: This Asian spice has become very popular in the West in recent years because of its enormous health benefits. It's known for reducing chronic inflammation in the body by blocking the chemicals that trigger inflammation to occur. Just a teaspoon of this spice is all you need to gain the benefits, and it adds a bright yellow color to your drinks! That's due to a pigment called curcumin that is found in turmeric.

✓ **Ginger:** This is another substance that reduces inflammation. It might not sound so tasty in a morning smoothie, but just adding a few small pieces of ginger can have a beneficial effect. Try and mix it with other strong ingredients, such as fruits that have natural sugars, or soy milk that can cover up the taste. You might have to do some experiments to find the right flavor balance, but don't leave this ingredient out!

✓ **Berries**: These are perfect for a smoothie and work naturally to fight inflammation in the body. Packed with natural antioxidants and tons of vitamins and minerals, there's so many for you to choose from depending on your favorite flavors! Blueberries, strawberries, raspberries... even cherries and pomegranate seeds are a great addition to any smoothie. And they're naturally sweet so you can cut back on any sugar you would have added!

✓ **Chia Seeds**: These little seeds have become the star in many dishes lately. Despite their size, they are packed with omega-3 fatty acids that work to combat inflammation in the body. By increasing the amount of fatty acids we eat, we can hopefully see inflammation reduce. Be sure to include a handful of these in your smoothie. They're mostly tasteless so you won't even know they're there!

✓ **Greens**: Spinach, kale, chard... yes, a green smoothie is synonymous with a healthy smoothie because it's the truth! They are high in antioxidants and enzymes that enter your bloodstream and break down molecules that cause inflammation. The more raw your greens are consumed, the more effective they are. Be sure to include a cup of greens in your smoothie is the best way to have your daily intake. Kale is considered a superfood because it is high in so many vitamins and minerals including riboflavin, iron, magnesium, and Vitamins A, K, B6, and C. Experiment with what combinations and amounts work best for you, and how you can combine them with a mix of other fruits and other vegetables.

✓ **Apples**: Though apples sometimes get looked over for other sweeter fruits, red apples have been researched and found to have antioxidants in their skin that act as a natural anti-inflammatory. Studies even found that people who eat three to five apples a week have a lower risk of developing asthma, which is an inflammatory condition. You can use green apples if you prefer the tartness, but don't forget some slices of apple in your smoothie to get all the nutrients!

✓ **Pineapples**: This delicious tropical fruit is rich in Vitamin C and an enzyme called bromelain. This enzyme digests other proteins, such as the ones that are causing trouble in the body by creating inflammation! It can reduce swelling, pain, and bruising in the body and give you arthritis and tendonitis relief. If you can find this fresh, it is a great addition to include in your smoothies - for the health benefits and the taste! If not, you can always find it canned but make sure you read the label and find the one with the least amount of artificial sugar.

✓ Nuts: When making your smoothie, be sure to add in a handful of nuts. Almonds are high in unsaturated fatty acids that work to keep the joints lubricated. Walnuts also contain similar fatty acids that release acids to protect the body from bone loss. Walnuts inhibit the production of neurotransmitters that cause pain and inflammation. Be sure that you are adding raw nuts and not a salty or sugary type.

✓ Kiwi: A fruit that's not paid too much attention to, recent research has shown that kiwis are packed with antioxidants and anti-inflammatory proteins. They are rich in fiber, vitamin E, potassium, vitamin K, and so many others! They are a tart and tangy fruit so if you can't eat it raw, it's great to include in your smoothies with other ingredients to balance or hide the flavor.

Here are some great recipes to get you started on making smoothies! The great thing about smoothies is that they are so versatile and it is easy to switch ingredients. If you don't prefer blueberries, try a different berry like blackberries. If you don't care for pistachios, try walnuts instead. These recipes are for making 1 serving so if you are having guests, feel free to double it!

Greek Yogurt Smoothie: This smoothie is filled with proteins, so it's perfect as a post-workout treat when the body is looking for proteins to rebuild muscle. It's also very filling so it can even replace dinner if you are trying to lose weight and maintain a healthier lifestyle. As mentioned, feel free to use whichever berries you prefer. Also, if you have another leafy green you like better, you can switch out the spinach for kale.

- 25 cup Greek yogurt, plain, no additives
- 1 cup nut milk, like cashew, almond, or soy
- 25 cup baby spinach

53

- 25 cup blueberries
- 2 tablespoons peanut butter
- 25 teaspoon of cinnamon
- a few ice cubes

Strawberry Red Smoothie: This smoothie is packed with sweet and tart ingredients that are packed with vitamins and minerals. The beautiful red color makes it already look delicious!

- 5 cup red beets, peeled and chopped
- a small half-inch piece of ginger, peeled
- 75 cup cranberry juice
- 75 cup strawberries
- a pinch of cinnamon
- 1 tablespoon organic honey
- a few ice cubes if you prefer!
-

Tropical Summer Smoothie: This smoothie is a beautiful yellow and is so delicious that you won't even remember how good it is for your health! With delicious tropical fruits, it's the best treat, especially on a hot summer day.

- 1 cup mango, fresh or frozen
- 1.5 cup cold water
- a few ice cubes
- 1 teaspoon turmeric
- a small half-inch piece of ginger, peeled
- 1 cup pineapple, fresh or frozen
- 5 teaspoon coconut oil

Sweet Potato Smoothie: Both spinach and sweet potatoes are healthy vegetables that can reduce inflammation. They're also a great source of magnesium. A magnesium deficiency can lead to muscle cramps.

- 5 cup sweet potato, cooked
- 5 cup almond milk
- 5 teaspoon vanilla extract
- a handful of baby spinach
- 1 teaspoon honey
- a pinch of cinnamon
- a small half-inch piece of ginger, peeled
- a half banana

Pineapple Turmeric Smoothie: Combined with turmeric and ginger, this fruit smoothie is a powerful tool to combat inflammation - and it's delicious! Try and find the freshest fruit you can, but if you can't, feel free to experiment with substitutes.

- a small half-inch piece of ginger, peeled
- 1 teaspoon turmeric
- 5 cup pineapple
- 5 cup mango
- 5 cup coconut milk
- 5 teaspoon vanilla extract
- a pinch of cardamom powder (or cinnamon, if you don't have it!)

Avocado Citrus Smoothie: Avocados are a superfood and contain high amounts of folic acid, vitamin C, vitamin E, and more than a dozen other nutrients! With some citrus fruit added as well, this smoothie is packed with tons of vitamin C.

- 1 avocado chopped into pieces
- juice of 1 small orange

- juice of 1 small lemon
- 5 teaspoon vanilla extract
- 1 cup milk of your choice
- 1 banana
- a few cubes of ice

Carrot Ginger Smoothie: Packed with tons of ingredients to combat inflammation, along with lots of Vitamin C, this smoothie is full of antioxidants and will fulfill some of your fruit and vegetable servings for the day.

- 5 cup cold water
- a small piece of ginger root
- juice of 1 small lemon
- 1 teaspoon turmeric
- 5 cup carrots, peeled and chopped
- 5 cup pineapple, fresh or frozen
- 5 cup milk of your choice
- 1 large ripe banana

Kiwi Ginger Smoothie: This smoothie shines on the healing power of kiwis that are believed to have anti-inflammatory proteins. It's a tangy fruit so feel free to add a handful of berries or a teaspoon of honey if you feel like you need to sweeten the flavor. Adding in nuts and gives you a boost of healthy fat and proteins too!

- 2 kiwis, peeled and chopped
- 1 ripe banana
- a small piece of ginger root
- 4 tablespoons cashews
- 5 cup water

- a few ice cubes
- 1 teaspoon of chia seeds

Strawberry Almond Smoothie: A simple smoothie consisting of berries and almonds, this is a great way to get your daily fruit intake, and some "good" fats with a handful of nuts! Almond milk is a great milk to use because it is packed with nutrients and gives more flavor than regular milk.

- 5 cup strawberries
- 1 cup almond milk, unsweetened
- 5 cup orange juice, natural
- 5 cup yogurt, no additives

Coconut and Ginger Smoothie: As we shared in the previous chapter, ginger is known for its medicinal anti-inflammatory properties. It can combat nausea, digestive issues, and believed to even stop the growth of cancer cells! This is a great and simple smoothie to have a healthy helping of ginger.

- 1 ripe banana
- 5 cup coconut milk
- a pinch of cinnamon
- a pinch of nutmeg
- 5-10 few pieces of ginger root, about an inch each, how many depends on how strong a flavor you like

Cucumber Pineapple Smoothie: Pineapples are high in bromelain which has been studied and found to inhibit inflammation and pain. With a hint of cinnamon to regulate blood sugar, this is a great treat of flavors.

- 5 cup pineapple chunks

- 2 small cucumbers, peeled and diced
- 5 teaspoon cinnamon powder
- 5 teaspoon turmeric powder

Blueberry Green Juice: This smoothie is just three ingredients but each one has unique properties to fight inflammation. Blueberries contain the most antioxidants compared to other fruits and vegetables, and spinach is high in folic acid!

- 1 cup blueberries, fresh or frozen
- 5 cup Fuji apples, peeled and chopped
- 1 cup fresh spinach leaves
- 5 cup cold water
- a few ice cubes

Watermelon Smoothie: This smoothie is perfect as a summertime treat. Even though watermelon is made up of mostly water, it's filled with a powerful antioxidant called lycopene. Lycopene works to protect the skin and internal organs and reduces inflammation in the body by neutralizing free radical ions. Other nutrients work to block the enzyme that causes pain and inflammation in the body. Be sure to pick the ripest watermelon you can find so you get all the nutrients you can!

- 3 cups watermelon, skin and seeds removed, cut into chunks
- 7-8 small basil leaves, fresh (use less if bigger size)
- juice of half a lime

Conclusion

Thank you for making it through to the end of *Arthritis Diet!* We hope that by reading this book some of your questions about arthritis and inflammation were answered. These are serious afflictions that millions of people live with on a daily basis, especially the elderly. Adjusting one's life to this disease and the constant swelling or pain accompanied with it can be devastating. Trying to maintain an active lifestyle if you had one before can become challenging. Whether you were simply looking for more information on these conditions or wondering about the causes for it, we hope this book has been informative in providing you answers. It's important to note that despite many potential causes of arthritis such as family history, lifestyle choices, and obesity, the majority of researchers believe that arthritis is a disease that the human body will eventually succumb to, no matter how healthy or active you are. That is simply how the human body is set up. Over time, the cartilage and joints begin to break down due to the body's weight and activities.

Before making any changes in your exercise or diet, you should speak to your primary care doctor regarding your arthritis pain. They may have other suggestions in mind or make you aware of any conflicts regarding medication you're taking. Making the switch to a vegan or vegetarian diet is also a big change and a doctor should be consulted.

If you're looking to make healthier choices in your diet and meals to ease arthritis symptoms and boost your immune system, we hope we've provided you with some great tips to get started. We've provided a great list of foods that you can incorporate more into your weekly menu. Foods like fish, beans, citrus fruits, and leafy green vegetables should be eaten a few times a week. Fruits and vegetables especially are very important, and if you can buy them organic, it's even better. Leafy vegetables like spinach and kale contain a variety of antioxidants that have been found to block the proteins that signal inflammation. Even adding just a little bit of minced garlic or ginger to your meals can be helpful too. And don't forget the olive oil! This oil is known to have medicine-like properties and should be used by arthritis patients in their meal preparation.

When talking about a healthier arthritis diet, it's also necessary to cut the processed, salty, or sugary snacks. It's especially important if you are trying to lose weight in order to ease your symptoms of arthritis. Excess weight puts pressure on the joints of the body and this stress speeds up the process of cartilage breaking down. Smoothies are a great way to pack many healthy ingredients into a drink, so you are getting as many nutrients as you can in the raw form. With the right ingredients, they can also be very filling and help you maintain a goal weight if you are struggling with meals. We've included nearly a dozen smoothie recipes so you can pick and choose the perfect treat for your flavor profile!

We hope that this book has given you some ideas on how to eat a healthier diet in hopes of reducing your pain and inflammation!

BONUS:

As a way of saying thank you for purchasing my book, please use your link below to claim your 3 FREE Cookbooks on Health, Fitness & Dieting Instantly

https://bit.ly/2EFv31x

You can also share your link with your friends and families whom you think that can benefit from the cookbooks or you can forward them the link as a gift!

:

Made in the USA
San Bernardino, CA
07 November 2019